Danielle Oliveira Maciel
Josiane Macedo de Oliveira Rupf
Elane Magalhães Oliveira

HIV/AIDS AND OPPORTUNISTIC INFECTIONS

Danielle Oliveira Maciel
Josiane Macedo de Oliveira Rupf
Elane Magalhães Oliveira

HIV/AIDS AND OPPORTUNISTIC INFECTIONS

A review of the literature

ScienciaScripts

Cover image: www.ingimage.com

This book is a translation from the original published under ISBN 978-613-9-68682-7.

Publisher:
Sciencia Scripts
is a trademark of
Dodo Books Indian Ocean Ltd. and OmniScriptum S.R.L publishing group

120 High Road, East Finchley, London, N2 9ED, United Kingdom
Str. Armeneasca 28/1, office 1, Chisinau MD-2012, Republic of Moldova, Europe
Printed at: see last page
ISBN: 978-620-8-31263-3

DANIELLE OLIVEIRA MACIEL JOSIANE MACEDO DE OLIVEIRA RUPF ELANE MAGALHÃES OLIVEIRA

HIV/AIDS AND OPPORTUNISTIC INFECTIONS: A LITERATURE REVIEW

SUMMARY

This paper aims to review the literature on HIV/Aids and associated opportunistic infections, emphasising the clinical relevance of these pathologies in immunosuppressed individuals.
The human immunodeficiency virus (HIV) progressively compromises the immune system, leading to the onset of acquired immunodeficiency syndrome (AIDS), at which point the body becomes vulnerable to a series of opportunistic infections. These infections are responsible for high morbidity and mortality rates among HIV+ patients, especially in regions with limited access to antiretroviral therapies. The review covers the main bacterial, viral, fungal and parasitic infections, including tuberculosis, pneumocystosis, cryptococcosis and toxoplasmosis, discussing their diagnosis, treatment and clinical implications. In addition, the impact of antiretroviral therapy on the prevention and control of these infections is analysed, as well as the challenges faced in treatment, such as drug resistance and lack of therapeutic adherence. The conclusion is that, although there have been significant advances in the management of HIV/Aids, opportunistic infections still represent a major challenge, especially in contexts of socio-economic vulnerability.

Keywords: *HIV, AIDS, opportunistic infections, antiretroviral therapy, tuberculosis*

SUMMARY

PART 1
INTRODUCTION

1 TOPIC UNDER STUDY

The human immunodeficiency virus (HIV) remains one of the most serious public health issues in the world, responsible for millions of deaths and infections over the last few decades. According to the World Health Organisation (WHO), in 2022, approximately 38.4 million people were living with HIV, and around 650,000 died from AIDS-related illnesses. HIV infection can lead to the development of Acquired Immune Deficiency Syndrome (AIDS), which occurs when the virus gradually compromises the immune system, leaving the body susceptible to a series of infections and diseases, often fatal, known as opportunistic infections.Opportunistic infections are caused by pathogens which, in people with a healthy immune system, are generally controlled by the body. However, in immunosuppressed individuals, such as those with HIV, these infections can manifest themselves in serious ways. Among the most common infections are tuberculosis, cryptococcosis and pneumocystosis, which represent a major clinical challenge. Tuberculosis, for example, is one of the main causes of death among people living with HIV, especially in developing countries. low and middle income, where health infrastructure is more precarious and access to adequate treatment is limited. The relationship between HIV and opportunistic infections was widely observed before the introduction of highly effective antiretroviral therapy (HAART), which drastically changed the prognosis of many patients. Before HAART, opportunistic infections were the main cause of death among people with AIDS. However, with the implementation of this therapy, it has been possible to drastically reduce the morbidity and mortality caused by these infections. HAART has enabled viral suppression and the recovery of the immune system in many cases, thus reducing patients' vulnerability to these infections. Studies show that since the introduction of HAART, there has been a considerable drop in deaths related to opportunistic infections, reflecting the effectiveness of the treatment.

Even with advances in treatment, opportunistic infections continue to be a concern, especially among those who do not have regular access to medication, receive a late diagnosis of HIV or have poor adherence to treatment. According to a systematic review conducted by Luma et al. (2013), adherence to antiretroviral therapy is crucial for preventing opportunistic infections. However, the lack of continuous access to medication in countries with weakened health systems remains a significant challenge, resulting in high mortality rates. Inadequate adherence to antiretroviral treatment can also facilitate the emergence of drug resistance, further complicating the situation for patients.

Among the most prevalent opportunistic infections in people with HIV/AIDS, tuberculosis occupies a central position and is responsible for a large number of deaths. According to UNAIDS data, tuberculosis remains the leading cause of death among people with HIV, and the risk of developing tuberculosis is 18 to 20 times higher in people with HIV than in the general population. This is due to the fact that HIV reduces the immune system's ability to fight infection, creating a favourable environment for the proliferation of Mycobacterium tuberculosis. Although there are effective treatments for tuberculosis, early diagnosis and proper management are essential to avoid fatal complications in people with HIV.

Another example of a relevant opportunistic infection is cryptococcosis, a fungal infection that mainly affects the brain and central nervous system of immunosuppressed people. Cryptococcosis is caused by the fungus

Cryptococcus neoformans, which can be found in environments such as soil and bird droppings. In people with HIV/Aids, cryptococcosis often manifests itself as cryptococcal meningitis, a potentially fatal condition if not treated in time. Treatment for this infection involves the use of potent antifungals, but as with other opportunistic infections, late diagnosis and limited access to medication can increase the risk of death.

Pneumocystosis, caused by Pneumocystis jirovecii, is another opportunistic infection common among people with HIV/Aids. This infection, which affects the lungs, can result in severe pneumonia and respiratory failure, and is one of the main causes of hospitalisation and death in immunocompromised people. Studies show that with the introduction of prophylaxis against pneumocystosis, there has been a significant drop in the incidence of this infection among people living with HIV, especially in those on antiretroviral treatment. However, in regions where access to these treatments is limited, pneumocystosis still poses a considerable threat to patients' health.

These examples illustrate the importance of early diagnosis and strict adherence to treatment to control opportunistic infections in people living with HIV/AIDS. The prevention of these infections depends heavily on access to antiretroviral therapy, which has the potential to suppress the HIV virus and strengthen the immune system, thus reducing the likelihood of opportunistic infections. In addition, it is continuous medical monitoring is necessary to identify and treat any signs of infection early on, ensuring better clinical outcomes for patients.

Although significant advances have been made in the management of HIV/AIDS and opportunistic infections, challenges remain, especially in low-income countries. Lack of health infrastructure, drug shortages and social stigmatisation are factors that still limit adequate access to treatment. Therefore, public policies that promote education, early diagnosis and the equitable distribution of medicines are key to tackling these obstacles and improving the quality of life of people living with HIV/AIDS.

In conclusion, HIV/AIDS and opportunistic infections remain a significant global health problem. Although antiretroviral therapy has provided important advances, the vulnerability of immunocompromised patients to opportunistic infections remains a major concern. The prevention and effective treatment of these infections requires a continued commitment to improving access to quality healthcare, HIV education and prevention strategies, and the elimination of social and economic barriers that still affect the most vulnerable populations.

2 BACKGROUND

The study of HIV/Aids and opportunistic infections is extremely relevant in the global public health scenario, considering the significant impact of these conditions on the mortality and morbidity of immunocompromised individuals. The HIV pandemic, which began in the 1980s, continues to pose a challenge, especially in low- and middle-income regions, where access to antiretroviral treatment (ART) and early diagnosis is limited. The emergence of opportunistic infections in people living with HIV/Aids is one of the main complications associated with the progression of the disease, and is responsible for a substantial proportion of AIDS-related deaths.

According to UNAIDS (2023), approximately 38 million people were living with HIV in 2022, and despite advances in antiretroviral therapy, around 650,000 deaths still occurred that year due to HIV/AIDS-related illnesses. Most of these deaths are associated with the failure of the immune system, which leaves room for opportunistic infections that, in healthy people, would rarely cause serious complications. This figure illustrates the magnitude of the problem and the need to further study ways of preventing and treating these infections in HIV-positive patients. positive. Infections such as tuberculosis, cryptococcosis, pneumocystosis and toxoplasmosis remain a major obstacle to the clinical management of individuals with HIV/Aids. Tuberculosis, for example, is considered the leading cause of death in people living with HIV, especially in low-income countries where HIV-TB co-infection is highly prevalent. As reported by the World Health Organisation (WHO, 2021), in 2020 around 214,000 people living with HIV died from tuberculosis, highlighting the deadly nature of this combination of diseases in regions with weakened health infrastructure.

Analysing opportunistic infections associated with HIV/Aids is essential for developing more effective public health strategies. In Brazil, the HIV/Aids epidemic has become increasingly concentrated in vulnerable populations, such as drug users, homeless people and LGBTQIA+ communities. These groups face greater difficulties in accessing adequate treatment and are often more susceptible to developing opportunistic infections. According to Garcia et al. (2018), stigma and social discrimination against people living with HIV/AIDS are still significant barriers to early diagnosis and proper treatment, which increases the risk of complications and disease progression for advanced stages.Antiretroviral therapy (ART) has transformed the history of HIV/Aids treatment, enabling patients to achieve a life expectancy similar to that of people without HIV, provided that diagnosis is made early and adherence to treatment is maintained. However, lack of adherence to treatment, especially in contexts of social vulnerability, and late diagnosis are factors that still contribute to the progression of HIV to AIDS and the emergence of opportunistic infections. Studies such as that by Luma et al. (2013) show that late diagnosis is associated with higher mortality rates due to complications caused by opportunistic infections.

This highlights the need for more effective interventions to ensure early diagnosis and adherence to treatment.

Another relevant aspect in the justification for this study is the economic and social impact of HIV/Aids and opportunistic infections. Individuals with HIV/Aids, especially when affected by opportunistic infections, often experience a significant decline in their quality of life, which impacts not only their physical health, but also their ability to work and maintain an active social life. As highlighted by Murray et al. (2020), opportunistic infections are among the main causes of prolonged hospitalisations in people living with HIV, which generates high rates of mortality. costs for health systems, especially in countries with limited resources.

In addition to the direct costs associated with treating opportunistic infections, such as medication and hospitalisations, there are also indirect costs, which include lost productivity, the burden on patients' families and the economic impact on public health systems. Studies by Jardim et al. (2019) indicate that in Latin America, the cost associated with treating a single opportunistic infection can be significantly higher than the cost of preventing these diseases through effective antiretroviral treatment and continued adherence to medical care. Therefore, this review of the literature on HIV/AIDS and opportunistic infections is justified by the need to better understand the interactions between the immunosuppression caused by HIV and the predisposition to develop these infections. By identifying the main challenges and advances in the treatment and prevention of these conditions, this study can contribute to the formulation of more effective public policies, improve clinical management and reduce HIV/AIDS-related morbidity and mortality rates. The review also becomes an essential resource for health professionals, researchers and policymakers seeking to address existing gaps in the prevention and treatment of opportunistic infections. Furthermore, the relevance of the topic increases when we consider recent advances in new technologies and treatment strategies. Current research into the use of vaccines, immunological therapies and new formulations of antiretroviral drugs brings hope that the impact of opportunistic infections could be further reduced in the coming years. Thus, this study not only reviews the knowledge accumulated to date, but also points to future research directions and interventions that could transform the public health scenario for people living with HIV. with HIV/Aids.

3 PROBLEMATISATION AND GUIDING QUESTIONS

The HIV/AIDS epidemic remains one of the main global public health concerns, despite significant advances in treatment, especially with the use of antiretroviral therapy (ART). However, opportunistic infections, which affect immunosuppressed individuals, still represent a critical challenge in the clinical management of the disease. These infections occur when the compromised immune system is unable to control pathogens that, under normal conditions, would not be so harmful. As a result, serious and often life-threatening complications arise. responsible for a high mortality rate among HIV patients who progress to AIDS. The literature points out that although ART has played a crucial role in reducing the incidence of many of these infections, the reality shows that factors such as unequal access to treatment, late diagnosis, poor adherence to therapy and drug resistance remain substantial barriers. In addition, the social stigma associated with HIV/AIDS in various parts of the world prevents many people from seeking adequate treatment or even obtaining an early diagnosis, exacerbating the problem. In low- and middle-income regions, where health systems are often underfunded and overburdened, the impact of these opportunistic infections is even more devastating.In this context, some fundamental research questions arise: How do opportunistic infections affect quality of life and mortality in people living with HIV/AIDS, even with the availability of ART? What are the main factors that hinder the early diagnosis and treatment of these infections? And finally, how can public health policies be improved to mitigate the impact of opportunistic infections on more vulnerable populations, especially in contexts of scarce resources and high social inequality? The first guiding question seeks to understand the direct impact of opportunistic infections on the morbidity and mortality of people living with HIV/Aids, especially in low-income regions. Evidence shows that even with the availability of ART, the progression of the disease can be accelerated by the occurrence of these infections, which worsen the clinical condition of patients. In addition, the quality of life of these people is profoundly affected, since many of these infections require prolonged hospitalisations and complex treatments. The second question explores the challenges associated with the diagnosis and treatment of opportunistic infections. Late diagnosis, difficulties in accessing appropriate treatment and drug resistance are obstacles that directly affect the effectiveness of treatment. The lack of infrastructure in health systems in developing countries, coupled with a shortage of financial resources, means that the treatment of these infections is often inadequate or non-existent.Finally, the third question seeks to investigate how public health policies can be improved to prevent and treat opportunistic infections in people living with HIV/AIDS. The need for early diagnosis, awareness campaigns and the equitable distribution of medicines are essential elements in reducing the incidence of these infections. Health policy reforms are crucial to ensure that the most vulnerable individuals have access to the care they need and that morbidity and mortality rates related to opportunistic infections can be effectively reduced.Therefore, the study of opportunistic infections in people living with HIV/AIDS is not only justified by the direct impact of these infections on patients' health, but also by the urgent need to review and strengthen public health strategies to deal with these challenges in a more effective and inclusive way.

4 OBJECTIVE GENERAL

To analyse the relationship between HIV/AIDS and opportunistic infections, highlighting the main clinical and epidemiological challenges in the diagnosis, treatment and prevention of these infections in people living with HIV, with the aim of identifying effective strategies to reduce the associated morbidity and mortality.

5 OBJECTIVES SPECIFIC

- Identify the most common opportunistic infections affecting people living with HIV/AIDS, analysing their prevalence and impact on disease progression.
- To assess the barriers faced in the early diagnosis and treatment of opportunistic infections, with an emphasis on low- and middle-income regions where access to healthcare is limited.
- To investigate the role of antiretroviral therapy (ART) in the prevention and control of opportunistic infections, analysing the effectiveness of treatment in different socio-economic contexts.
- To propose improvements in public health policies aimed at the prevention and treatment of opportunistic infections, suggesting strategies that guarantee greater access to treatment and early diagnosis, especially for vulnerable populations.

PART 2

THEORETICAL FRAMEWORK

6 HISTORY AND EVOLUTION OF HIV/AIDS

The HIV/Aids epidemic began in the early 1980s, when the first cases began to be reported in the United States. Initially, the disease seemed like a new immunosuppressive condition with no defined cause, which alarmed the medical community due to its rapid progression and severity in young, healthy and mostly homosexual men. In 1981, the US Centers for Disease Control and Prevention (CDC) published the first official report describing cases of Pneumocystis jirovecii pneumonia and Kaposi's sarcoma affecting immunosuppressed individuals, marking the beginning of the identification of what would later be known as Acquired Immune Deficiency Syndrome (AIDS). According to Sharp and Hahn (2011), the human immunodeficiency virus (HIV), which causes AIDS, originated from a zoonotic transmission between chimpanzees and humans in Central Africa, and is related to the simian immunodeficiency virus (SIV).In the early years of the epidemic, the lack of knowledge and social stigma surrounding AIDS slowed down the global response to the crisis. The disease quickly came to be associated with marginalised groups, such as homosexuals and drug users and sex workers, which fuelled prejudice and hindered public awareness. According to Fee and Krieger (1993), the social stigma associated with AIDS contributed to governments and health systems being slow to implement prevention and treatment campaigns. Between 1981 and 1985, the number of cases continued to rise exponentially, becoming a real global public health crisis. It wasn't until 1983 that researchers at the Pasteur Institute in France, led by Luc Montagnier, identified the virus that causes the disease, HIV. The isolation of the virus was a milestone in the fight against the epidemic, as it enabled the development of diagnostic tests and paved the way for research into possible treatments. Shortly afterwards, in 1984, Robert Gallo in the United States also identified HIV as the causative agent of AIDS, confirming the previous findings. From then on, it became possible to detect HIV in infected people even before AIDS developed, a breakthrough that, although significant, did not bring an immediate solution for controlling the disease. In the absence of effective treatment, AIDS continued to spread devastatingly. By the late 1980s and early 1990s, the disease had reached pandemic proportions, affecting millions of people around the world. The impact was particularly severe in sub-Saharan Africa, where HIV infection rates were extremely high. According to Piot et al. (2001), the international response to the epidemic was slow and fragmented, and many low-income countries faced difficulties in implementing effective prevention programmes due to a lack of resources and the social stigma surrounding the disease.

The turning point in the fight against HIV/Aids began in the second half of the 1990s, with the development of antiretroviral therapy (ART). In 1996, a combination of antiretroviral drugs, known as a cocktail, proved to be effective in suppressing HIV replication, allowing patients' immune systems to recover and preventing the progression of AIDS. According to Deeks et al. (2015), ART transformed HIV from a fatal disease into a manageable chronic condition, provided treatment was started early and followed continuously. From that point on, the life expectancy of people living with HIV increased considerably, especially in countries where access to treatment was guaranteed.

However, challenges remain. Although access to ART has been expanded in many countries, millions of people in low- and middle-income regions still face difficulties in obtaining adequate treatment. The Joint United Nations Programme on HIV/AIDS (UNAIDS) estimates that, by 2022, around 38 million people were living with HIV worldwide, and more than 650,000 people have died as a result of AIDS-related illnesses. Late diagnosis, poor adherence to treatment and unequal access to health services continue to be the main obstacles to controlling the epidemic. Another important aspect of the evolution of HIV/Aids is related to awareness and prevention campaigns, which have played a crucial role in reducing the rates of new infections. Promoting the use of condoms, sex education and rapid testing programmes have been essential in halting the spread of the virus, especially in regions where the epidemic has reached alarming levels. According to the WHO (2020), pre-exposure prophylaxis (PrEP) has also become an effective tool in HIV prevention, especially for populations most at risk, such as men who have sex with men, injecting drug users and sex workers.

In recent years, scientific progress has brought new hope. Studies into a functional cure for HIV, which involves strategies to eliminate or significantly reduce the presence of the virus in the body without the need for ongoing medication, have advanced. In addition, HIV vaccines are being developed and tested in clinical trials, although none have been approved to date. Fauci and Marston (2015) emphasise that although a definitive cure is still a long way off, advances in research offer prospects promising for the future. Thus, the history and evolution of HIV/Aids reflects both the enormous challenges faced by global society and the significant advances in medical science. Although there is still no definitive cure, the development of ART and new prevention strategies has transformed the epidemic, allowing millions of people to live long and productive lives. However, it is crucial that the global community continues to invest in research, access to treatment and public health policies in order to achieve complete control of the epidemic and, eventually, the eradication of HIV.

7 OPPORTUNISTIC INFECTIONS IN PATIENTS WITH HIV/AIDS

Opportunistic infections are one of the biggest threats to patients living with HIV/AIDS, especially those who do not have access to adequate treatment or who have poor adherence to antiretroviral therapy (ART). These infections occur when the immune system is severely compromised by the HIV virus, which makes the body vulnerable to pathogens that would not normally cause illness in individuals with a healthy immune system. According to Kaplan et al. (2009), opportunistic infections are responsible for for a significant part of morbidity and mortality among people with AIDS, causing serious and often fatal complications.These infections occur because HIV destroys CD4+ cells, which play a crucial role in the body's defence against infections. As the count of these cells decreases, the body's ability to fight pathogens is reduced, allowing opportunistic infections to take hold. When the CD4+ cell count falls below 200 cells/mm³, the risk of these infections increases significantly, marking the transition from HIV-positive status to AIDS. Hoffmann and Rockstroh (2012) emphasise that in advanced stages of immunosuppression, the body becomes vulnerable to a series of infections that can be fatal if not treated properly.Among the most common opportunistic infections in HIV/AIDS patients is tuberculosis (TB), which is one of the main causes of death among these individuals. According to the World Health Organisation (WHO), people living with HIV are 18 times more likely to develop TB than the general population. HIV-TB co-infection is particularly prevalent in low- and middle-income countries, where living conditions and access to adequate health services are limited. In addition to tuberculosis, other bacterial infections, such as bacterial pneumonia and septicaemia, are also common. frequent among immunocompromised patients, resulting in prolonged hospitalisations and high treatment costs.Another common opportunistic infection is pneumocystosis, caused by the fungus Pneumocystis jirovecii, which mainly affects the lungs, causing severe pneumonia. This condition was one of the main causes of death in AIDS patients before the introduction of ART. Although prophylaxis with antiretroviral drugs has reduced the incidence of pneumocystosis, it still poses a significant threat in regions where access to ART is limited or where HIV is diagnosed late.Cryptococcosis, another fungal infection, is also common in people with AIDS and is caused by the fungus Cryptococcus neoformans. This infection usually manifests itself as cryptococcal meningitis, an inflammation of the membranes surrounding the brain and spinal cord. Without proper treatment, cryptococcosis can be fatal in a short period of time. It is estimated that, globally, more than 220,000 cases of cryptococcal meningitis occur annually among people living with HIV, resulting in around 180,000 deaths, as reported by Park et al. (2009).In addition to bacterial and fungal infections, parasitic infections such as toxoplasmosis are also prevalent in HIV/Aids patients. Toxoplasmosis is caused by the parasite Toxoplasma gondii and, in immunocompromised people, it can causes encephalitis, a serious inflammation of the brain. According to studies, cerebral toxoplasmosis is one of the main neurological opportunistic infections in AIDS patients and is associated with symptoms such as seizures, headaches and neurological deficits. Treatment for toxoplasmosis is complex and requires a combination of anti-parasitic drugs, and early diagnosis is crucial to avoid serious complications. Cytomegalovirosis, a viral infection caused by cytomegalovirus (CMV), is also commonly seen in HIV/Aids patients, mainly affecting the eyes, gastrointestinal tract and lungs. In immunocompromised individuals, CMV can cause retinitis, an inflammation of the retina that can lead to blindness, as well as severe pneumonia and colitis. Like other opportunistic infections, the incidence of cytomegalovirus has been reduced with the advent of ART, but it remains a significant problem in patients with advanced HIV who do not receive adequate treatment.The control of opportunistic infections depends largely on the effective use of antiretroviral therapy, which suppresses HIV replication and allows the immune system to partially recover. When treatment is started early and followed consistently, the risk of opportunistic infections is drastically reduced. However, in many parts of the worldwide, especially in low- and middle-income countries, access to antiretroviral drugs is still limited, and many patients are only diagnosed with HIV in advanced stages of the disease, when they are already severely immunosuppressed and vulnerable to opportunistic infections. In addition to the challenges of access to treatment, poor adherence to ART is a frequent problem, especially in vulnerable populations such as injecting drug users and homeless people. As Luma et al. (2013) point out, inadequate adherence to treatment not only increases the risk of HIV progression to AIDS, but also facilitates the development of drug resistance, making the control of opportunistic infections even more difficult. Raising awareness about the importance of adherence to treatment, combined with public policies that guarantee equitable access to healthcare, are essential to combat opportunistic infections in people living with HIV/AIDS.In conclusion, opportunistic infections continue to be one of the main causes of complications and death among people with HIV/AIDS, despite advances in antiretroviral treatment. Although ART has significantly reduced the incidence of these infections, challenges related to access to treatment, late diagnosis and inadequate adherence still prevent many people from benefiting fully from medical advances. Effective management of these infections requires not only an accessible and effective health system, but also a continuous effort to educate the population about the importance of early diagnosis and adherence to treatment, especially in more vulnerable regions.

8 ANTIRETROVIRAL THERAPY AND THE CONTROL OF OPPORTUNISTIC INFECTIONS

A antiretroviral therapy (ART) represents one of the most significant advances in the treatment of HIV/Aids, having radically transformed the way the disease is managed. Introduced in the 1990s, ART, which consists of a combination of drugs that inhibit the replication of HIV in the body, has the main objective of preventing continuous damage to the immune system, preventing or delaying the development of AIDS. With the effective use of ART, it is possible to keep the viral load undetectable, allowing the immune system to recover and function properly. This, in turn, drastically reduces the risk of developing opportunistic infections, which are one of the main causes of serious complications and deaths among people living with HIV. One of the main benefits of ART is its ability to prevent opportunistic infections, which arise when the immune system is weakened. HIV destroys CD4+ cells, which are essential for fighting infections. When the count of these cells falls below 200 cells/mm³, the body becomes highly vulnerable to a series of infections that, in healthy individuals, would be easily controlled. By suppressing the replication of HIV, ART allows the CD4+ cell count to rise. increases and is maintained at levels that guarantee protection against opportunistic pathogens. According to Lawn et al. (2017), ART is highly effective in preventing infections such as tuberculosis, pneumocystosis and cryptococcosis, all opportunistic infections common among people living with HIV who do not receive adequate treatment.

As well as preventing the emergence of new opportunistic infections, ART also plays a fundamental role in controlling infections that are already present in patients with advanced HIV. Patients who start antiretroviral therapy with a severely compromised immune system can nevertheless experience a significant improvement in their immune response, which can help control active infections such as Pneumocystis jirovecii pneumonia and cerebral toxoplasmosis. According to Deeks et al. (2015), many patients who start ART even in advanced stages of the disease show a significant recovery in their CD4+ cell count, which allows them to fight pre-existing infections.

ART also has a direct impact on reducing HIV/AIDS-related mortality. Before the introduction of this therapy, opportunistic infections were the main cause of death among people living with HIV, and were responsible for a high rate of hospitalisation and serious complications. Studies such as that by Palella et al. (1998) indicate that, since the implementation of ART, there has been a reduction of more than 80 per cent in HIV/AIDS-related deaths, with a large part of this reduction attributed to the prevention and effective treatment of opportunistic infections.

However, the success of ART depends on its continuous administration and high adherence to treatment. In many low- and middle-income countries, access to ART is limited, and adherence to treatment can be hampered by factors such as social stigma, lack of resources and difficulty accessing health services. Patients who do not strictly adhere to ART run the risk of seeing the HIV virus become resistant to the drugs, which not only makes it difficult to control viral replication, but also increases the likelihood of developing opportunistic infections. Poor adherence to treatment can therefore reverse the advances made with ART and put patients at high risk of serious complications.

Another important aspect related to ART is the role of therapy in low-income settings, where drug availability and health infrastructure are often insufficient to meet demand. In many of these contexts, opportunistic infections continue to be a significant cause of death among people living with HIV. Luma et al. (2013) point out that in areas where access to ART is limited, opportunistic infections continue to be a significant cause of death among people living with HIV. represent a major challenge for the management of the disease. In these cases, interventions that guarantee equitable access to ART, combined with prevention strategies, are fundamental to reducing HIV/AIDS-related mortality.In short, antiretroviral therapy plays a central role in controlling opportunistic infections in people living with HIV/AIDS. By restoring immune function, ART not only prevents the emergence of these infections, but also helps to control those already present in patients who start treatment at advanced stages of the disease. Despite the significant advances made with ART, challenges such as access to treatment and continued adherence remain critical, especially in low-income contexts. Therefore, the continued success of ART depends on global efforts to guarantee universal access to treatment and public health policies that promote education and support for patients living with HIV.

9 SOCIO-ECONOMIC CHALLENGES AND THE MANAGEMENT OF OPPORTUNISTIC INFECTIONS

The management of opportunistic infections in people living with HIV/AIDS is deeply linked to various socio-economic factors, which directly influence the evolution of the disease and the effectiveness of treatments. Although the advent of antiretroviral therapy (ART) has transformed the course of HIV/AIDS, significantly improving the quality of life and life expectancy of patients, socioeconomic barriers continue to hamper access to essential health care, aggravating the impact of opportunistic infections, especially in low- and middle-income countries.

Limited access to quality health services is one of the main challenges faced by patients living with HIV, especially in low-income regions. In many countries in sub-Saharan Africa and in low-income areas in Latin America and Asia, the healthcare infrastructure is insufficient to meet the demand for treatment for HIV and its complications. According to the

UNAIDS report (2021), around 10 million people worldwide living with HIV still do not have access to antiretroviral therapy, which significantly increases the risk of opportunistic infections and AIDS-related complications. This lack of access is exacerbated by the shortage of qualified health professionals, inadequate medical equipment and the lack of availability of essential medicines for the treatment of both HIV and opportunistic infections. In addition, in countries with few resources, geographical barriers and the high cost of treatment make it even more difficult to access the necessary care. Many patients living in rural or remote areas are unable to access regular This results in late diagnosis and progression of the disease without adequate treatment. These patients are particularly vulnerable to serious opportunistic infections such as tuberculosis, pneumocystosis and cryptococcal meningitis, since their weakened immune system is unable to fight these pathogens.

Another major challenge in the management of HIV/Aids and opportunistic infections is social stigma and discrimination. Prejudice around HIV/AIDS is still a reality in many parts of the world, preventing many people from seeking early diagnosis and treatment. According to Nguyen et al. (2018), social stigma causes many to avoid health services, which results in less HIV testing and more diagnoses in advanced stages of the disease, when opportunistic infections are already present and severe. This prejudice also affects the professional lives of patients, who often face discrimination at work and are forced to hide their status to avoid being marginalised. This discrimination directly impacts their ability to hold down a stable job, jeopardising their income and, consequently, their access to necessary medical care. Lack of financial resources makes these individuals even more vulnerable, especially in contexts where the costs of medicines and treatments are high.In addition, unequal access to ART is another problem. critical factor. Although ART has revolutionised HIV/Aids treatment, enabling many patients to live long and healthy lives, access to this treatment is still profoundly unequal, especially in low- and middle-income countries. While in developed countries the introduction of ART has been accompanied by a sharp drop in HIV-related mortality and complications associated with opportunistic infections, in poorer countries the implementation of this therapy has been limited by a lack of funding, inadequate infrastructure and logistical difficulties. According to Luma et al. (2013), these barriers mean that many patients only have access to treatment when they are already in advanced stages of the disease, which limits the benefits of ART and increases the risk of serious complications, including opportunistic infections.

Therefore, tackling opportunistic infections in people living with HIV/Aids goes beyond the medical control of the disease and requires a broad approach that takes into account the socio-economic challenges that affect access to treatment and early diagnosis. Overcoming these challenges involves implementing public policies that guarantee equitable access to healthcare, reducing social stigma and promoting HIV/AIDS prevention and awareness programmes, especially among the most vulnerable populations. Only with a global effort coordinated, it will be possible to mitigate the impact of opportunistic infections and improve the quality of life of people living with HIV/AIDS around the world.

PART 3
REFERENCE METHODOLOGICAL

10 TYPE OF RESEARCH

This work adopts a bibliographical research methodological approach, characterised by the analysis of secondary data, with the aim of identifying, describing and discussing the main information available in academic literature on the subject of "HIV/Aids and Opportunistic Infections". Bibliographic research is widely used in review studies, as it allows the exploration and integration of various sources of knowledge, including scientific articles, books, reports from health organisations and other relevant documents, offering a solid basis for the discussion and interpretation of the phenomena under study.

According to Gil (2008), bibliographical research seeks to understand the state of the art of a given topic by gathering information that has already been published, organising it and interpreting it critically. In the present study, bibliographical research was selected as the central method for the literature review, since the chosen theme involves analysing data and existing information on the impact of opportunistic infections in people living with HIV/AIDS and the effectiveness of antiretroviral therapy (ART) in controlling these infections.

The choice of this type of research is justified by the vast scientific production available on the subject, which includes empirical studies, systematic reviews and reference documents from organisations such as the World Health Organisation (WHO) and the Joint United Nations Programme on HIV/AIDS (UNAIDS). In this way, the literature search provides a comprehensive and up-to-date overview of opportunistic infections in HIV-positive patients, as well as the socio-economic challenges and therapeutic solutions related to the management of the disease.The methodology used for data collection included searching academic databases such as PubMed, SciELO, Google Scholar and VHL (Virtual Health Library), as well as reviewing scientific articles published in indexed journals of high relevance in the field of public health and HIV/Aids. To ensure that the information was relevant and up-to-date, publications from the last five years were prioritised, except in the case of fundamental texts that deal with concepts or classic studies on the subject.In addition to the bibliographical research, clinical practice guidelines and public health policies will be considered, as will provide an applied and practical perspective for understanding the management of opportunistic infections in the context of HIV/AIDS. The data will be analysed qualitatively, with a focus on identifying patterns, gaps and innovations in the treatment and prevention practices of these infections, especially with regard to the implementation of ART in different socio-economic contexts.Therefore, the bibliographical research adopted in this work will enable a broad reflection on the subject and will contribute to building a critical understanding of the central issues related to HIV/Aids and opportunistic infections, based on evidence consolidated by scientific literature.

11 PLACE AND PERIOD OF RESEARCH

This literature review study was conducted using secondary data sources, without the need for a specific physical location to collect the information. The research was based on materials available in online academic databases such as PubMed, SciELO, Google Scholar and the Virtual Health Library (VHL), which provide access to a wide range of scientific articles, books, health reports and institutional publications relevant to the topic being addressed. In this way, the research site comprises the virtual environment, which offers vast access to global scientific production on HIV/AIDS and opportunistic infections. The research period was from September 2023 to October 2023. During this period, scientific articles, systematic reviews, clinical practice guidelines and reports from public health organisations such as the World Health Organization (WHO) and the Joint United Nations Programme on HIV/AIDS (UNAIDS) were collected and analysed. The choice of this period is justified by the need to gather recent and up-to-date data, prioritising publications from the last five years, except when it was necessary to include older reference works for the theoretical development of the topic. The review was conducted with a focus on understanding the strategies for controlling opportunistic infections in people living with HIV/AIDS and the impact of antiretroviral therapy (ART), as well as identifying the socioeconomic challenges that influence access to treatment.

12 PARTICIPANTS IN THE SURVEY

As this research is bibliographical in nature, there is no direct participation by individuals or groups of people. Instead, the "participants" are the authors and the studies included in the literature review. Bibliographic research involves analysing and interpreting scientific articles, books, reports and guidelines from public health institutions, published by various sources. specialists in the fields of HIV/AIDS, opportunistic infections and antiretroviral therapy (ART). The studies analysed were selected based on criteria of relevance, with priority being given to papers published between 2018 and 2023, in order to ensure that the information used is up-to-date and reflects the current state of research and clinical practice in the treatment of HIV/AIDS patients. In addition, classic texts on the subject were also considered to support essential concepts. The main authors and institutions whose work was reviewed include renowned researchers and organisations such as the World Health Organisation (WHO), the Joint United Nations Programme on HIV/AIDS (UNAIDS) and other global reference bodies in the field of public health.This approach allows for a comprehensive understanding of the subject based on a variety of reliable and scientifically validated sources.

13 INCLUSION CRITERIA

The inclusion criteria adopted in this bibliographic research were established to ensure the relevance, timeliness and quality of the information analysed. The first criterion considered the period of publication, with priority given to studies published between 2018 and 2023, in order to guarantee that the data and information used was up to date. However, studies from before this period were included when they were considered fundamental to understanding the historical and theoretical development of HIV and opportunistic infections.

The second criterion involved selecting recognised academic and scientific sources. Only articles published in journals indexed in reliable databases such as PubMed, SciELO, Google Scholar and the Virtual Health Library (VHL) were used. In addition, reports from renowned international organisations such as the World Health Organisation (WHO) and the Joint United Nations Programme on HIV/AIDS (UNAIDS) were included as valid sources to guarantee the consistency and credibility of the information. The third criterion focussed on thematic relevance, with the inclusion of only studies that directly addressed the central theme of the research, i.e. HIV/Aids, opportunistic infections and antiretroviral therapy (ART). The research focused on the clinical and socio-economic challenges involved in controlling these infections in HIV-positive patients.Another essential criterion was the rigorous methodology of the selected studies. Only studies that presented methodological clarity, well-defined objectives and detailed analyses were included. Systematic reviews and meta- High-quality analyses were prioritised in order to provide a comprehensive and reliable overview of the subject.Finally, it was necessary for the studies to be available in full text, so that all the relevant information could be accessed and analysed properly, guaranteeing the depth and integrity of the research carried out. These inclusion criteria were fundamental in ensuring that the literature review offered a solid, comprehensive and reliable basis, allowing for a critical and well-founded analysis of the topic.

14 EXCLUSION CRITERIA

The exclusion criteria adopted in this research were defined to ensure the relevance and quality of the sources used to analyse the topic of "HIV/Aids and Opportunistic Infections". The first criterion established was the exclusion of publications prior to 2018, except in cases where they were considered fundamental to the historical or theoretical understanding of the evolution of HIV treatment and opportunistic infections. This ensured that the information was up-to-date and reflected the current state of science. In addition, sources other than scientific rigour, such as blogs, popular media reports or websites without peer review. Only academic articles and scientifically validated publications were included, ensuring the credibility and quality of the information analysed. Studies with inadequate methodologies, unclear design or superficial analyses were also discarded. The exclusion of these studies aimed to ensure that the research was based on consistent and well-founded data.

Another exclusion criterion was incomplete access to articles. Publications that required payment or were available only as abstracts or previews were disregarded, since access to the full text is essential for a detailed and critical analysis of the information. In addition, articles that did not directly address the topic of HIV/AIDS, opportunistic infections or antiretroviral therapy (ART) were excluded. Only papers that dealt with clinical, epidemiological or socio-economic aspects related to the topic were considered.

Finally, studies that presented outdated or decontextualised data in relation to the current understanding of the epidemiology and treatment of HIV/Aids and opportunistic infections were also excluded. In this way, the exclusion criteria adopted allowed the research to be conducted on the basis of relevant, up-to-date and high quality sources. quality, guaranteeing a critical and consistent analysis of the subject.

15 INSTRUMENT FOR COLLECTING DATA

In this bibliographical research, the data collection tool used was a systematic literature review. This instrument consists of searching for, selecting and analysing relevant scientific publications on the subject of "HIV/AIDS and Opportunistic Infections". The collection process was carried out by consulting academic databases such as PubMed, SciELO, Google Scholar and the Virtual Health Library (VHL), which provide access to scientific articles, books, reports from public health institutions and systematic reviews.

The search strategy included the use of keywords such as "HIV", "AIDS", "opportunistic infections", "antiretroviral therapy" and "ART", combined with Boolean operators ("AND", "OR") to ensure that the most relevant and specific studies were found. Filters were also applied to the databases to restrict the search to publications from the last five years, prioritising the most recent, except when it was necessary to include historical or classic studies that were fundamental to the topic.

After the initial search, articles were screened based on the defined inclusion and exclusion criteria previously. The full text of the selected articles was analysed qualitatively, focusing on identifying relevant information for the discussion on the impact of opportunistic infections in HIV/AIDS patients and the effectiveness of antiretroviral therapy in controlling these infections.Thus, the data collection tool was a review and critical analysis of the available scientific literature, with the aim of consolidating current knowledge on the subject and offering a comprehensive and grounded view of the clinical and socio-economic challenges related to HIV/Aids and opportunistic infections.

16 PROCEDURES FOR COLLECTING DATA

The data collection procedures for this bibliographical research followed a systematic and organised approach, with the aim of ensuring that relevant information was obtained from reliable sources. The first step was to select the main academic databases, where searches were carried out for scientific articles and publications on the subject of "HIV/Aids and Opportunistic Infections". The databases chosen were PubMed, SciELO, Google Scholar and the Virtual Health Library (VHL), recognised for their vast availability of peer-reviewed studies of high scientific quality. Once the databases had been defined, the keywords that guided the search, such as "HIV", "AIDS", "opportunistic infections", "antiretroviral therapy" and "ART". These words were combined using Boolean operators such as "AND" and "OR" in order to expand or refine the results, ensuring that the most relevant studies to the topic were included in the search. Filters were then applied to the databases to restrict the results to recent publications, i.e. those published between

2018 and 2023, ensuring that the information analysed was up-to-date and reflected the most current scientific knowledge. Exceptions to this criterion were made only for classic or fundamental studies for the historical and theoretical understanding of the subject. After the initial search, the articles found were screened based on the previously defined inclusion and exclusion criteria. This screening involved reading the titles and abstracts and, when necessary, consulting the full text to determine the relevance of each study to the topic. The selected articles were then read and analysed in detail. The main focus of this stage was to identify the most relevant information on the impact of opportunistic infections on HIV-positive patients, the effectiveness of antiretroviral therapy in controlling these infections and the socio-economic challenges associated with treatment. The information extracted from the studies was recorded in an organised manner, categorising the main points discussed in each publication, such as the authors, objectives, methodology and results. This process The data recording system served as the basis for summarising and discussing the information presented throughout the work. With these procedures, data collection was carried out carefully, using reliable, up-to-date and scientifically validated sources, providing a solid basis for analysing the subject of "HIV/Aids and Opportunistic Infections".

17 ANALYSING DATA

The data in this bibliographical research was analysed qualitatively, based on a review and critical interpretation of selected publications on the subject of "HIV/Aids and Opportunistic Infections". The main objective was to identify patterns, discuss the clinical and socio-economic challenges related to these infections in people living with HIV and assess the effectiveness of antiretroviral therapy (ART) in controlling these complications. The data collected was organised into central themes, such as the prevalence of different opportunistic infections, the impact of ART in preventing these infections and the socio-economic challenges that hinder access to treatment and control in different contexts. The analysis revealed that opportunistic infections continue to be one of the main causes of morbidity and mortality. mortality among people with HIV/AIDS, especially in low- and middle-income countries. Tuberculosis, for example, is one of the most common infections among HIV-positive patients, especially in regions with poor health infrastructure. According to the World Health Organisation (WHO), people living with HIV are up to 20 times more likely to develop tuberculosis, especially in places where access to ART and other health services is limited. This emphasises the importance of public health policies aimed at expanding access to ART in these regions.Another important aspect identified in the analysis is the role of ART in reducing opportunistic infections. By increasing the CD4+ cell count and improving the immune response, ART has been fundamental in preventing and controlling these infections. In countries where ART is widely accessible, the rate of opportunistic infections has fallen significantly. However, factors such as lack of adherence to treatment, difficulty accessing drugs and late diagnosis remain critical challenges, especially among more vulnerable populations. These obstacles limit the effectiveness of ART and increase the risk of serious complications related to opportunistic infections. The analysis also showed that socio-economic inequalities play a decisive role in the prevalence of these infections. Regions with the greatest disparities People with low incomes and less access to health services face greater challenges in controlling HIV/AIDS and opportunistic infections. Social stigma, discrimination, geographical distance to health services and the high cost of treatment are barriers that hinder adequate access to ART and the effective management of these infections. In conclusion, the data analysed reinforces the importance of interventions that improve access to ART and promote adherence to treatment, as well as implementing public policies that reduce inequalities in access to health services. Although ART has made considerable progress in controlling opportunistic infections, the socio-economic context and social stigma remain major challenges, especially in the most vulnerable populations.

18 RISKS OF RESEARCH

This research, which is bibliographical in nature, does not involve direct interaction with human beings, which eliminates physical, emotional or psychological risks, since there is no collection of primary data or field experiments. However, there are some risks inherent in this type of study, which can affect the quality and validity of the results.

One of the main risks is related to the limitation of data sources. Bibliographic research depends on the quality, quantity and accessibility of the studies available in databases. As pointed out by Gil (2008), one of the limitations of this type of research is the possibility that the literature selected does not completely cover the topic, which can compromise the breadth of the analysis. If the search for relevant literature is not sufficiently comprehensive or up-to-date, there is a risk of leaving out recent and relevant studies, especially in an area that is constantly evolving, such as the treatment of HIV/Aids and opportunistic infections. Another risk is selection bias, which occurs when the researcher chooses studies that may reflect personal preferences or results that corroborate their initial hypothesis. According to Pereira et al. (2013), selection bias is a concern in bibliographic research, since it can influence the objectivity of the analysis and lead to biased conclusions. To mitigate this risk, the research used strict and clearly defined inclusion and exclusion criteria, prioritising the inclusion of studies of high relevance and scientific rigour, published in recognised sources such as indexed databases.

The research also faces the risk of subjective interpretation of the data, since qualitative analysis depends on the researcher's interpretation when synthesising and evaluating the information obtained. According to Lakatos and Marconi (2017), subjectivity in qualitative analysis can be a limitation if there is no robust theoretical foundation and careful comparison between findings. To reduce this risk, multiple reliable sources and comparisons between different approaches were used, ensuring a balanced and critical view of the subject studied. Therefore, although the risks are minimal, the limitations of bibliographical research, such as the restriction of data sources, selection bias and subjective interpretation, were managed with methodological rigour, guaranteeing the quality and reliability of the results presented.

PART 4
RESULTS AND DISCUSSION

The research, bibliographical in nature, presents risks However, it is not without some of the limitations inherent to this type of study. One of the main risks is the limitation of data sources, which can compromise the scope of the analysis. According to Gil (2008), bibliographic research depends entirely on the quality and quantity of publications available, which can restrict the depth of the investigation if the sources are limited or out of date. As scientific literature is constantly evolving, especially in the field of HIV/Aids, the absence of recent studies can result in outdated conclusions.Another important risk is selection bias, which can occur if the researcher chooses specific subsets of the literature, reflecting personal preferences or confirming previous hypotheses. According to Pereira et al. (2013), selection bias in bibliographic research can negatively influence the objectivity of the results, since the studies selected may not reflect the diversity of approaches and perspectives required for a complete analysis. To avoid this risk, strict inclusion and exclusion criteria were adopted, and the screening process was carefully carried out to ensure that only studies of high quality and relevance were considered.

Furthermore, the risk of subjective interpretation is a concern in qualitative analyses, as the synthesis of the data depends on the researcher's interpretation. Lakatos and Marconi (2017) point out that subjectivity can introduce bias into the analysis, especially if the researcher does not apply a critical approach when comparing findings from different sources. To mitigate this risk, a critical and rigorous approach was used, ensuring that multiple sources were analysed and compared, thus guaranteeing a balanced interpretation of the data. Thus, although there are risks related to the limitation of sources, selection bias and subjectivity in the interpretation of data, these factors have been minimised through a well-defined methodology and the use of strict criteria. As a result, the research offers a reliable and well-founded analysis on the subject of "HIV/Aids and Opportunistic Infections".

CONCLUSION

This bibliographical research allowed for a comprehensive analysis of the impact of HIV/Aids and opportunistic infections, highlighting the importance of antiretroviral therapy (ART) in preventing these infections and improving patients' quality of life. From the literature review, it became clear that although ART has revolutionised HIV treatment, significantly reducing morbidity and mortality, opportunistic infections still represent a major problem. great challenge, especially in contexts of socio-economic vulnerability.The research showed that unequal access to ART, lack of adherence to treatment and late diagnosis are factors that contribute to the persistence of opportunistic infections such as tuberculosis, pneumocystosis and cryptococcosis. These problems are more prevalent in low- and middle-income countries, where health infrastructure is limited and the stigma surrounding HIV/AIDS prevents many people from seeking proper treatment. In addition, socio-economic challenges such as poverty, lack of access to health services and discrimination are significant barriers to the effective control of these infections. Analysing the data reinforces the need for more inclusive public policies that guarantee equitable access to ART and promote adherence to treatment, as well as initiatives to combat the social stigma associated with HIV.Therefore, it can be concluded that, despite advances in the treatment of HIV/AIDS, opportunistic infections continue to represent a significant risk for people living with the disease, particularly in less favoured regions. Increased access to ART, health education and the reduction of socio-economic inequalities are essential in order to improve the management of these infections and reduce their impact on global public health. Continued commitment to these interventions will be key to tackling the challenges that still exist in controlling HIV/AIDS and opportunistic infections.

REFERENCES

GIL, Antonio Carlos. **Social Research Methods and Techniques** 6. ed. São Paulo: Atlas, 2008.

HOFFMANN, Christian; ROCKSTROH, Jürgen K. **HIV Medicine .** Oxford: Flying Publisher, 2012.

Portuguese KAPLAN, JE; BENSON, C.; BROOKS, JT **Guidelines for the prevention and treatment of opportunistic infections in HIV-infected adults and adolescents .** MMWR Recomm Rep, v. 58, p. 1-207, 2009.

LAKATOS, Eva Maria; MARCONI, Marina de Andrade. **Fundamentals of Scientific Methodology .** 7. ed. São Paulo: Atlas, 2017.

LAWN, SD; MEINTJES, G.; MCILLERON, H.; WOOD, R.

Management of HIV-associated tuberculosis in resource-limited settings: a state-of-the-art review . BMC Medicine, v. 11, p. 253, 2017.

LUMA, Henry; DOUMBOUYA, A.; SOPIAGNE, A.; MIMBOUE,

E. **Late presentation for HIV/AIDS treatment in Douala General Hospital: prevalence, predictors and implications for mortality . International Journal of STD & AIDS, v. 24, p. 293-297, 2013.**

NGUYEN, Vinh-Kim; STENGEL, Ellen. **The political economy of HIV: how HIV/AIDS interventions have shaped global health and development .** Global Health, v. 14, p. 2, 2018.

PEREIRA, Andreia; SANTOS, Maria José; LOPES, Patrícia. **Literature Review:** Steps and Success Factors . Acta Médica Portuguesa, v.26, p. 255-258, 2013.

UNAIDS. Global statistics on HIV and AIDS - **Fact sheet .** 2021. Available at: https ://www .unaids .org /en /resources /fact -sheet . Accessed on: 10 October 2023.

WORLD HEALTH ORGANISATION (OMS). **HIV /AIDS :**

Key facts . 2020. Available at: https://www.who.int/news-room/fact-sheets/detail/hiv-aids . Accessed on: 10 Oct . 2023 .

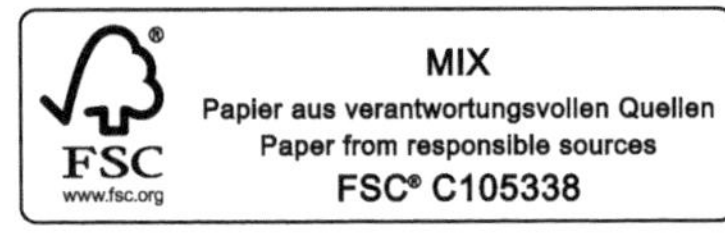

Printed by Books on Demand GmbH, Norderstedt / Germany